I0789163

<u>*Also by Dr. Stenbeck*</u>

<u>*Available from the usual on-line source*</u>

<u>*Books*</u>
Healing Yourself -- The Holistic Approach
  [An introduction to Holistic Self-healing.]

Heal Yourself Right Now!
  [The Seven Priority Organ Levels for
  effective Nutritional/Holistic Treatment of
  all organs.]

The 22 Unique Body Types
  (for Health and Weight Loss)

Q & A to Identify Your Body Type (Booklet)
  [Individual Type booklets are also available

<u>*Booklets*</u>
(Step-by-step instructions on healing yourself)

  #1 Start Healing with Positive <u>Thinking</u>
  #2 Mastering Positive <u>Feelings</u> for Health!
  #3 <u>Spiritual</u> Balance and Your Healing

The Desmogenic Body Type

Representing one of the 22 Body Types first described by Victor Rocine around 1900

The Daniel Craig, Tina Turner Celebrity Body Type

*For Kaye,
there at the beginning with Doc Severn,
and for Liberty,
continuing the holistic healing journey…*

About the Author

Educated in New Zealand and in the U.S.A., Dr. Stenbeck attained B.Sc. (NZ), M.S., and D.C. degrees. His holistic healing methods have been profiled in magazines (Esquire, McLean's, Playgirl, the Atlanta Constitution), and on TV in the USA and in Canada. He was the main contributor to the Warner Book, *The Eye/Body Connection* by Jessica Maxwell that focused on the holistic healing relationships between the iris structure and organ genetics.

In the 1970-80's he was elected Fellow, Royal Society of Health, London; Fellow, American

Association of Chemists; Member, American Association of Clinical Chemists; and Affiliate, Royal Society of Medicine, London. He studied naturopathy and Body Types with Dr. Bernard Jensen and Dr. Clifford Severn, and has practiced in medical partnerships where patients received the joint benefits of medical and holistic healing.

He is a member of Self-Realization Fellowship. To receive advice on any health issue from a holistic viewpoint, or to receive help with your body type, see his web site: *DrStenbeck.net*

———

Contents

***

The Desmogenic Body Type
(and Food Guide) 1

***

The 22 Body Types: Celebrity Examples

This Booklet contains the **Desmogenc** *type. [See* <u>The 22 Unique Body Types</u> *for all type descriptions.]*

Thin Types

Atrophic   Woody Allen / Audrey Hepburn
             Stan Laurel / Calista Flockheart

Exesthesic Cher / Sarah Jessica Parker
             (Female type only)

Marasmic   President Obama / Princess Diana
             James Stewart / Kate Blanchard

Neurogenic J.K. Simmons / Joan Rivers
             Jon Cryer / Marin Hinle

Pathoferic (No celebrity males)
             Blythe Danner / Gwyneth Paltrow

Sillevitic David Bowie / Shirley MacLaine
             Rod Stewart / Carol Channing

Muscle Types

Calciferic *Michael Jordan / Angelica Huston*
      Abraham Lincoln / Grace Jones

Carbogenic *George Clooney / Lady Gaga*
      Pres. G. Bush, Jr. / Meg Ryan

Desmogenic *Marlon Brando / Loni Anderson*
      Daniel Craig / Tina Turner

Eldic   *Ross Perot / Hillary Clinton*
      Peter Falk / Sigourney Weaver

Medeic   *David Caruso/Madonna*
      John Hurt / Marlene Deitrich

Myogenic *Pres. Bill Clinton / Sharon Stone*
      Pres. John Kennedy / Julia Roberts

Nervimotive *Frank Sinatra / Elizabeth Taylor*

Nitropheric *Ben Affleck / Ava Gardner*
      Kirk Douglas / Kate Winslet

Pallinomic *Pres. Donald Trump /*
      Attorney General Janet Reno
      Bill O'Reilly (Fox) / Jane Russell

Fat Types

Barotic — *Robin Williams / 'Mrs.Doubtfire'*
Elton John / William Conrad

Carboferic — *Bill Murray / Roseanne*
Billy Gardell / Melissa McCarthy

Hydripheric — *John Goodman / Shelly Winters*
Wayne Knight / Jennifer Holliday

Isogenic — *Einstein / Oprah Winfrey*
Phillip S .Hoffman / Queen Victoria

Lipopheric — *Rush Limbaugh / Rosie O'Donnell*
Chris Christie / Camryn Manheim

Oxypheric — *Winston Churchill / Orsen Welles*
Ella Fitzgerald / Gerry Spence

Pargenic — *Burt Reynolds / Katey Segal*
Ron Perlman / Kirstey Alley

<u>Succinct Quote on Human Types</u>

From Victor Rocine, who first described discrete body types around 1900.

"A type is an order of people that differentiates and distinguishes itself by a general and similar form, brain-formation, chemistry, structure, build, immunity, tendencies, predisposition, resemblance, skin-pigment, and type characteristics based on observation and analogy.

"Or, in other words, people of a given type are similar physically and like-minded as if they were brothers and sisters—that is what type means.

"Everything in nature is made according to plan. Man only discovers that plan and gives it a name. The zoologist has not made the animals—he has only described the plan adopted by the wonderful Creator, and named the classes, sub-classes, etc.

"How important type research will be to humanity, time alone will make known."

———

Prologue

The esteemed scientist J. J. Berzelius, discoverer of several chemical elements, inspired Victor Rocine to research body types and to investigate the correlation between types and their diseases. Around 1890-1910, Rocine privately published his original findings on the mineral basis of different body types, and this present book exists because of his brilliant insights.

For many years, I studied with Dr. Clifford Severn who had been a personal student of Victor Rocine on body types, naturopathy, herbology, iris analysis, diet, and nutritional healing methods. He had a successful career as a lecturer and healer, and was one of those rare athletes with complete muscle control over his body. I saw him under a spotlight at 85 years of age, contracting and rippling every individual muscle in his perfectly developed body. Field-Marshal Jan Smuts, the WWII South African Prime Minister, devoted a full chapter of his autobiography to how Severn's healing methods had saved his life. In the 1950's, *Life* magazine did a four-page spread on Severn and his family. Fame he had.

Another Rocine student I studied with, Dr. Bernard Jensen wrote of Rocine's body type research and nutritional methods in his privately published book *The Chemistry of Man.*

This book is deeply rooted in Rocine's original work, and with that of Herbert Shelton, M.D., Ph.D. (at Harvard University in the 1930's). I integrated their research with newer dietary and nervous system data along with celebrity examples of each type, hopefully, making this material easier to digest and more entertaining for the reader.

Gayelord Hauser, another Rocine student I knew, was a celebrated health book author. He wrote a popular book on Rocine's types in the 1940's, *Types and Temperaments;* reputedly, he also introduced yogurt to the western world.

This book exists because of Rocine's creative brilliance and original discoveries in natural healing.

▶ *Rocine: "The soul creates the body type."*

Rocine taught that the soul chooses a body type and brain to live in, thus presenting different experiences and life lessons to master. Why were *you* born the way you are?

That is something to think about, especially if it is true! What would your soul purpose be to live in a particular body type. I provide some thoughts on this issue in each type description and try to assess from my experience with your type the particular lessons of life presented therein.

Rocine was as brilliant in his way as an Abraham Lincoln, Michael Jordan, Michael Phelps, Tony Robbins, or a Daniel Day Lewis—all *calciferic* types—rare, leaders, innovative, brilliant, and highly intelligent in their different fields of endeavor.

Celebrity examples exist for most types, not a duplicate of you, but someone who has your essence in their body-mind individuality. Knowing your type allows you to become a better you!

The celebrity examples provide further help in identifying your body type.

▶ *Rocine's classic findings are the backbone of this book. Integrated with Sheldon's research and with other dietary and food issues including mental, emotional, and spiritual attributes,*

Many people take nutritional supplements and try different diets without a doctor's advice. If this is your choice, use common sense, listen to body responses, and discontinue any allergic reactions to foods or nutritional substances.

———

The Desmogenic Body Type

Representing one of the 22 Body Types first described by Victor ʀᴏᴄɪɴᴇ around 1900

"*You may also have a physical or psychological feature not representative of your type such as height, weight, appearance, talent, weakness, strength, etc., due to biochemical errors, environmental influences, racial or cultural differences, and congenital or genetic issues. Nevertheless, the type identification of the average person is usually clear.*"

— *Victor Rocine*

Desmogenic Type Celebrity Examples

If you think this is your type, be sure to look at **on-line photographs** *of these examples. Look for general similarities to yourself. Note that sub-types cause the differences in appearance between members of the same type.*

GOVERNMENT

President Vladimin Putin
President Gorbachev (and most
    Russian Premiers)
    Madeleine Albright (Secretary of State)
    Barry Goldwater
    House Speaker Newt Gingrich
    Governor Ann Richards
    General Al Haig Jr.
    Congressman Bob Dornan

MILITARY

General George S. Patton (WW II)
(You are very attracted to the military and police as professions: you are warriors and leaders.)

ACTORS

Daniel Craig	Marlon Brando
Richard Burton	Robert Shaw
Val Kilmer	Albert Finney
Richard Harris	Tony Danza
Oliver Reed	Yul Brunner
Rod Steiger	Jack Lord
Michael Pare	

Loni Anderson	Dyan Cannon
Joan Crawford	Carol Lawrence
Gloria Swanson	Tina Louise

TV

Roma Downey	Pamela Anderson
Anna Nicole Smith	Della Reese

VOICE (Many singers of this type)

Tony Bennett	Tom Jones
Engelbert Humperdinck	
Tina Turner	Carol Lawrence
Reba McIntire	Cleo Lane (jazz)
Bonnie Raitt	

SPORTS

George Foreman	Evander Holyfield
Mike Tyson	

Joe Frazier   Bo Jackson
Dennis Rodman
Jim Brown
Joe Louis (and many professional boxers)
Many boxers, professional athletes, football
owners and coaches.
Serena Williams

ARTS/OTHER

Miles Davis   Elvin Jones
                              (Drummer)

RELIGION

Oral Roberts   Jimmy Swaggart
Kenneth Copeland   Martin L. King, Jr.

HISTORY (from Rocine)

Beethoven   Houdini

[I knew two of the above celebrities, and numerous examples in everyday life, which contributed to my understanding of the type.]

You already know something about this type from their public persona and appearance, whether from seeing them yourself or from the celebrity examples. Blend such insights with the type descriptions and the types of your family and friends to discern their presence in your midst!

Read the types, and if still confused you may choose to use the personal request for type identification from my web site: *DrStenbeck.net*

5

Desmogenic Type Questionnaire

These questions describe the generic type, and not specifically you! If any question ever applied to you, then choose the True answer!

For question 1 only:

A = True	*B = Maybe*	*C = Untrue*
15 points	*7 points*	*1 point*

1. Physically identify with celebrity example ____

Then…

A = True	*B = Maybe*	*C = Untrue*
5 points	*3 points*	*1 point*

---

2. Height is close to:
   Males: 5'6-5'11   Females: 5'4-5'9   ____
3. Usual weight is close to:
   Males: 160-280+   Females: 155-190+   ____
4. Body medium-sized when younger;
   often heavier after age 30 (with a fat
   sub-type you may become obese)   ____
5. Muscles extremely strong (males)   ____
6. Mentally and emotionally intense:
   think, feel, and act with conviction   ____
7. Always ready to take action   ____
8. Prominent cheek bones, sunken cheeks;
   muscular wide chin (males especially)   ____

9. Face wide between the ears and at angles of the jaw, markedly in some men; less-so in females   _____

10. Skin attractive if healthy; with aging, females may have yellow-white skin deposits under the eyes; some males may have pock marks following acne (*pargenics* also)   _____

11. Teeth white, strong when young: may yellow older age   _____

12. Some social or excessive drinkers; some abstain alcohol   _____

13. Sides of face are vertical on frontal view   _____

14 Hair dark, bushy, strong in youth, grays easily (females often dye hair blonde); often thin or balding hair by age 30-40   _____

15. Males: light chest hair; females medium to large bust   _____

16. Smoke cigarettes (or used to)   _____

17. Have genuine courage; fearless in face of the enemy; are born leaders   _____

18. Desire to be in control, in command   _____

19. Non-magnetic personality; rule by domination and control   _____

20. Not liked as bosses, make others uncomfortable   _____

21. History of joint pains or arthritis   _____

22. Are strong carnivores, crave flesh; difficult to be vegetarian   _____

23. Strong sexual drive and needs   _____

24. If wronged, some are vindictive and
    take revenge   _____
25. Intense likes, dislikes, beliefs   _____
26. Rebellious nature from early childhood _____
27. Opinionated, suspicious, accusative   _____
28. Are combative   _____
29. Never retreat from any position,
    physical or intellectual   _____
30. Many singers; voice is strong, resilient;
    some males have a high-pitched voice   _____
31. Vain: first in line for face-lifts,
    anti-aging remedies   _____
32. Have a blistering temper   _____
33. Body resilient, powerful, athletic,
    attractive   _____
34. High intellect and intelligence; honest
    forceful opinions   _____
35. Often cold, stern, forceful, and striking
    appearance; men handsome; females
    attractive, may be beautiful   _____
36. May become heavy with age (from a
    fat sub-type)   _____
37. Head large above and behind ears;
    wide temples; forehead may be large
    in central section   _____
38. Eyes commanding; eyebrows straight,
    eyes hypnotic   _____
39. Ears may be set lower on head;
    hearing is exceptional   _____
40. Some crave alcohol, tobacco, sex,
    exercise, hallucinogens   _____

41. Effective weight-lifters; may gain
    great strength ____
42. Fine skin wrinkles; perspire easily ____
43. Dimpled chin characteristic in males,
    less-so in females ____
44. Upper lip thin and firm: lower lip
    larger, fuller often blue-red color ____
45. Nervous and restless disposition ____
46. May be extreme, reactive, demanding,
    unpredictable ____
47. Muscles compact, like 'steel springs',
    may be great athletes ____
48. Positive one day, negative the next ____
49. Arms, legs, fingers muscular, powerful ____
50. Strong bones and joints until arthritic ____
51. Back strong and muscular; shoulders
    square and broad ____
52. Intense nerves, emotions, thoughts ____
53. Speak truth bluntly and honestly ____
54. Bold, big risk-takers (hence are
    successes or failures) ____
55. Ambitious, keaders, achieve power ____
56. Love freedom, truth, independence ____
57. Never retreat mentally or physically;
    will literally die before giving in ____
58. May be changeable, moody, depressed ____
59. Strongly rebellious and combative ____
60. Never intimidated (intimidate others!) ____
61. Are watchful, observant, controlled
    until aroused verbally or physically ____
62. Naturally aggressive; need to 'step
    down' to assertiveness ____

63. Are bad boys and girls at school   _____
64. Not warm, friendly or magnetic; cool, detached, and solitary   _____

Scoring

For Question #1:

A response: give 15 points   = _______
B response: give 7 points   = _______
C response: give 1 points   = _______

For Questions #2—64:

A response: give 5 points   = _______
B response: give 3 points   = _______
C response: give 1 point   = _______

Total of the above points   = _______

Interpretation

160—300: PROBABLY Desmogenic

84—159: POSSIBLY Desmogenic type

<84: NOT Desmogenic type

The Desmogenic Type

Rocine: "Desmogenic means 'banded ligaments for bone and joint strength.' You are <u>the</u> sodium type." You are often deficient in food sodium, which is essential for your healing.

You have a natural musculature, a medium-build, medium-height or shorter (never tall), and are handsome and attractive or beautiful. When young, your tissues are flexible, tight, and compact, giving you a lean, resilient, wiry, muscular, shapely, attractive, and powerful body, which allows you to be dancers and professional or Olympic athletes. The salt-shaker and salted foods contribute to your disease processes.

Your weight may increase with age in both sexes unless carefully eating and exercising. The older males may stand out with their bony bald skull (or hairpiece), and a muscular-fatty build. Older attractive females, often fat or matronly with white or blonde hair, are usually of your type. (If more plain looking, you are more likely to be a *pallinomic* type.)

Both sexes show great mental and emotional intensity, a determined stubbornness, and an ability to "move mountains with the mind." You may be stern, cold, threatening, or striking in demeanor.

▶ *Rocine: "You have great gifts of mind and body, and potentially have a superior intellect and intelligence. Honest and forceful expression of opinions characterizes your personality."*

You are as lithe as cats and similar to the tiger and leopard in strength, style, speed, and grace. You are born to bravery and leadership, as seen in the great battlefield Generals George Patton, Erwin Rommel. and most German and Russian generals of WWII. (Note that British and U.S. Generals were predominantly the *nitropheric* type with *desmogenic* sub-types.) There are many excellent examples in the police and military.

Often found in politics, your brain and ego propel you to success, conservative Newt Gingrich being a good example.

► *The following statement by former Speaker Newt Gingrich is so typical of this type. He describes himself as:*

> *"I'm the sort of guy who goes into a room and breaks furniture. I'm very high tempo: a high–risk offensive coach. I want to get things done. I want to take risks."*

[A perfect description of the type from one of its members!]

Along with the *carbogenic and nervimotive* males, you are willing to "push the edge of the envelope until you succeed."

———

Physical Similarity to Other Types

The *myogenic* type (Christopher Reeve, JFK) is muscular, but more gentle, open, and approachable compared to the average *desmogenic.*

The *nitropheric* type (Gregory Peck, Kim Novak) is often shapely and attractive like the *desmogenic,* but is more demure, laid-back, and peaceful. Many times *nitropherics* have a *desmogenic* sub-type, making it difficult to differentiate physically between them. But, the personalities are so different!

The *carbogenic* type (Hugh Jackman, Sally Field) is shapely and attractive, but has more hair, is mostly calm and peaceful, and is usually taller.

———

Average Height and Weight

Males:	5'6-5'11	160-280+ pounds
Females:	5'4-5'9	155-190+ pounds

Note that you are very rarely tall. More often you are of medium height, or shorter.

———

Desmogenic Type Description

The type description represents how you appear in everyday society. You may have a sub-type that alters parts of this description.

Think of the celebrity examples as you read the descriptions. You gain weight if not exercising and eating sensibly; conversely, by taking care of yourself you may remain lithe and attractive throughout life. Your weight may increase with aging, and obesity occurs in those with a fat sub-type like Marlon Brando. Some of you, with aging, retain your hair and your handsome or lovely figures and beauty. When around this type you will experience their emotional intensity in everyday life.

Two distinct varieties of your type:
- One of medium-height, with longer arms and legs (Daniel Craig)
- A shorter, more wiry and stocky example with immense strength (in boxers like Mike Tyson, and in many Olympic athletes)

The strongest male and female body-builders in the world with their rippling muscles are of your type.

▶ *Rocine: "You are the most physically powerful and emotionally intense type on earth. The calciferic is the most powerful mental person."*

Head — Your head has wide temples, large above and behind the ears, and the forehead may be large.

Hair —Dark, bushy, stiff, strong, and healthy hair is typical when younger; the males have a balding tendency from about age 30, although many of the females also lose their hair. A famous celebrity I knew, had fabulous hair, until she took it off! The main balding types are the *desmogenic, neurogenic, pargenic, and calciferic.*

Eyes — Your eyes are mostly gray, green, or blue, and may seem cold and commanding. People say "you are able to stare right through them." Straight eyebrows, sunken eyes, an intense gaze makes you great hypnotists. You see better in the dark, and are sensitive to strong light.

Ears — The ears are set lower on the head, and your sense of hearing is exceptional.

Nose — A muscular nose with an acute sense of smell is common; as soldiers you may scent the enemy.

Face — Your prominent cheekbones, sunken cheeks and muscular chin are distinctive.

► *The angles of your jaw are often wide or pointed (but less so in many females). In other types, this jaw feature indicates a desmogenic sub-type.*

On frontal view the classic *desmogenic* face is wide between the ears, straight up and down on the sides, with pointed angles of the jaw. A dimpled chin is characteristic in many mesomorphs. Note that the Kennedy brothers and Jacqueline Kennedy Onassis are *myogenics* with very pointed angles of the jaw; in them, this feature indicates a *desmogenic* sub-type. It is noteworthy that the *desmogenic* sub-type is very common in other muscle types.

Mouth and Lips —Your upper lip tends to be thin and firm; the lower is large and full, and may have a darker cast. Your voice is strong, sometimes squeaky in men, and you may be a dynamic speaker.

Teeth — Strong and white teeth are typical; teeth deterioration and yellowing may occur, with age, from food sodium and potassium deficiencies.

Skin —Your complexion is pale looking with fine wrinkles, and you perspire easily.

▶ *Rocine: "Colored deposits in the skin, under the eyes, occur in middle-age females commonly due to excessive uptake of beta carotene, and excess bile production."*

Neck —A short, strong, and inflexible neck is common.

Muscles — Your compact lithe muscles, more obvious in the males, are as strong as steel springs. You enjoy intense exercising. The gyms are full of your type, and you are born for sports and athletics: the harder it is the better you like it, and eventually some of you wear out your body.

Chest — You have a prominent and strong chest; the bust is medium-sized or large. Males have a light growth of chest and body hair, although some have a hairy chest and body (due to *carbogenic, nervimotive, or pargenic* sub-types).

Back and Shoulders —Your back is strong and muscular, the shoulders square, broad, muscular, and powerful.

Hips and Abdomen —The hips and abdomen are narrow, flat, and muscular until middle-age when you usually spread out.

Arms and Legs — The arms are lean, muscular, powerful, while the legs are heavier; you may have short arms and legs; long palms, short and strong fingers; the fingernails may bend inwards.

Joints — Powerful, strong and yielding joints are common; your bones do not break easily, but the males are quite capable of breaking other peoples' bones! However, you often suffer with arthritis and metabolism problems due to sodium excesses, potassium deficiency, and toxic metal issues.

———

Desmogenic Personality Traits

If you are this Muscle type many, but not all, of the following characteristics are present—you may have overcome or moderated the negatives, but recognize that you once had several of them.

You may have any of the following traits:

- Love of nature
- Are somewhat nomadic
- Forcefully express opinions
- Are devoted to those you love
- Are great athletes, boxers, wrestlers
- Are achievers, roll-over all resistance
- Great endurance, tenacity and intuition
- Possessed of a sharp and pointed intellect
- Feel better in the mornings, worse at night
- Act with speed, grace, precision, efficiency
- May crave spicy foods, meats, alcohol, drugs

- Ambitious and achieve power and leadership

▶ *Rocine: "You are bold and big risk-takers (hence you are great achievers or great failures). You are the most emotionally intense of all types."*

- Have a wonderful mind, but some are very lazy
- Are the best guards, warriors, policemen, soldiers
- Some like consulting with psychics and astrologers
- Difficult, demanding, and intimidating (do it my way)
- Highly passionate with intense feelings and behaviors
- Handshake may be crushing (unaware of own strength)
- Desire freedom, truth, independence, and being in command
- Nerve intensity, muscle strength, mental coolness in emergencies
- Generally skeptical of orthodox religions (some start their own religion)
- Are watchful, observant and controlled, but if aroused express vocal and physical power

- Not warm, friendly or magnetic like *myogenics*; in fact, you are often disliked for your emotional intensity

———

Potential Challenges

▶ *Rocine: "You are the most intense of all people!"*

If you relate to any of these challenges, doing something to overcome them serves your evolution. You may have evolved from or have not experienced these general challenges, so don't dwell on this list. Note that any *desmogenic* may be calm, polite, gentle, spiritual, and I have known examples to be this way; however, some of you have many of the following aspects.

▶ *Rocine: "You never retreat from a mental or physical position: you die before giving in. You cannot surrender. This makes for impossible arguments with your loved ones: you cannot allow another person to win a point—with wisdom you allow that others may also be right!"*

- Highly intense, opinionated
- Many are jealous and controlling

- May exploit the weaknesses of others
- Nervous intensity may drive others away
- May have peculiar moods, depressions, recklessness
- Nobody can disrupt your positive opinion of yourself
- Some, may become manic, jealous, shameless, vindictive
- Are often suspicious, scornful, accusative, intolerant, jealous
- You often have arrogant self-confidence and self-superiority
- Aggression predominates: you may need "anger management"
- Tendency to radicalism or religious extremes (many TV evangelists)
- You are often unforgiving if crossed; some vindictive and revengeful
- Intense feelings of rebellion, combativeness, physical prowess, etc., propel some of you into crime
- Exercise addiction is common in males (who may physically damage themselves through forceful exercise)
- You may be critical, outspoken, sarcastic, and undiplomatic; you make enemies easily (but also have many friends and followers)
- Rebellious nature; you invariably had a troubled childhood; may have brushes

with the law over assaults, theft, or sexual abuse

- Disobedience is an instinctive behavior; males may be expelled from schools in formative years; your anger may be uncontrollable
  [Nevertheless, you may consider all of the above to be strengths.]

▶ *Rocine: "You may react in a blistering and scathing manner until your lips, nerves and muscles tremble, and your feelings explode."*

[He was describing your type from over 100 years ago, but many of you have the potential to react in this way.]

———

Desmogenic Stress Management

Your *mental and emotional* stress prevention is strong, giving you a good ability to prevent stress internalization.

———

Love

You are particularly attracted to the *carbogenic, carboferic, eldic, exesthesic, myogenic, nitropheric, and neurogenic* types. Your sexual drive is intense from a young age, and masturbation or sexual activity may occur before age 10. When in love, you may be devoted, possessive, and jealous—the males, particularly, may claim ownership of a person (like some *carbogenic* men who are more charming).

———

Talents and Vocations

Abilities - *Military, authoritative, executive, police, sports, business, investments*

The *desmogenic* is happiest when independent and in command, obvious careers being the military and police where your tenacity and talents propel you through the ranks; you make excellent officers and detectives; you crave the adrenalin of threat and danger.

► *I have known or observed you as boxers, lawyers, executives, orchestral conductors, retired millionaires, racing car drivers, air force fighter pilots, actors and talent agents, coaches and gym instructors, professional and Olympic athletes, and many in real estate (especially females) and in business.*

You, and the *carbogenic* type, are the elite of professional athletes as champions in boxing, baseball, karate, wrestling, contact sports, and football (most running backs). Other professions attracting you are athletic coaches in high school, college, and professional sports. You also make tough and effective executives. The type information cannot predict what or who you will become, but you are capable of bringing a creative excellence or brilliance to whatever you do in life.

Inabilities - *Arts, compassionate human relations*

You rarely have occupations requiring sensitive human interaction and artistic pursuits, although I know a few who are artistic, successful, and emotionally and spiritually evolved.

———

Health Problems

You become sick easily, but like the "cat with nine lives" you live them to the fullest! You crave fatty meats and excessively absorb protein, salt and sodium foods leading to bone, joint and connective tissue problems. When sick, you commonly experience health problems or diseases in any of the following organs and tissues:

Gastro-intestinal System — Stress internalized into your digestive tract causes health problems.

Heart, Lungs, Circulation — You become diseased from smoking, drugs, alcohol, and from over-eating fatty meats.

Muscles — Generalized muscle pains are common, and you may feel worse after exercise. Some are extremists, and may exercise yourselves into the grave.

Chronic Infections — You may suffer from hoarseness and chronic infections (teeth, gums, rectum, bladder, etc.).

Fat — If not careful, especially if you have a fat sub-type, your weight increases dramatically after age 30-40; you need exercise and dieting.

Bones, Joints, Ligaments — There is a strong tendency to arthritis, gout, cartilaginous, fibrous and ligament problems; you suffer from more gout than any other type, and should avoid common salt.

▶ *If arthritic, Rocine recommends a high food sodium vegetable broth of potato peelings; this high source of food sodium helps keep calcium in solution and out of your joints.*

———

Desmogenic Acid/Alkaline Factor

For your health and healing, the genetics of your autonomic nervous system predispose you to needing a specific ratio of food acidity to alkalinity. You are born with an *alkaline* constitution, which means you need a predominantly **acid-ash** food intake for acid/alkaline balance. (Ash refers to the minerals left in your body after metabolizing foods.) Your autonomic nervous system genetics are *parasympathetic* dominant, theoretically needing 70% *acid-ash* foods (proteins, carbohydrates) in your diet, but...

> *For your healing, if in ill health or after about age 40-45, you need to aim for this approximate ratio of food selections:*
> *50% Fruits, salads, vegetables*
> *50% Proteins, carbohydrates*

Some of you choose to become vegetarians, but be sure to take a daily protein drink (in addition to protein and carbohydrate foods). If you avoid flesh eat more acid-ash foods like carbohydrate vegetables (yams, squash, potatoes, pumpkin, etc.), and vegetarian proteins, spirulina, etc.

▶ *Approximate your food ratios. On any particular day, it does not matter if one meal is mostly alkaline and another mostly acid—just try to balance it out for the day! If you make a mistake, try again tomorrow. It is a subjective call that you make, as what you do over weeks and months makes the difference to your health.*

The Desmogenic Spiritual Factor

Skip this paragraph if uninterested in a philosophical perspective on your type!

▶ *Rocine: "The soul chooses the body type."*

· If as souls, we choose the brain and body type to spend a lifetime in, it could be to learn certain spiritual lessons related to perfecting ourselves, and our humanity, in God's eyes. What lessons does the type bring you? Only you can really decide what those lessons are. You know your weaknesses and faults, and what goes through your head, and how you behave towards others. You know things about yourself that Victor Rocine could never get his research subjects to say. Each discrete type has challenges of life lessons, spiritual goals, etc., and some of yours may be:

Faith — You need a relationship with a loving God, and once attained, you believe intensely in God.

Rebellious — Your middle names are rebellion and disobedience: give yourself permission to conform a little.

Emotional Intensity — Potentially, you may be angry and intense; if so, you need therapeutic help to keep this excessive emotion under control and not to hurt others. You may have an obvious propensity to acting out with anger, rage, fury, or destructiveness, particularly with people who don't agree with you or who interfere with what you are doing.

Opinionated — You are unendingly forceful with outspoken and sarcastic opinions: learn to get along with people. (But then again, you may not care to.)

———

A Desmogenic Story...

Muriel, age 49, was beginning to look matronly. Her type tendency of gaining weight had been manageable until age 35-40 when it went out of control. She was also concerned about her worsening temper and aggressive way of dealing with her friends and family. Her built-in anger and aggression with people moderated with therapy and a correct diet.

Examination revealed the typical food abuses of her type with excessive intake of these carbon and sodium junk foods: carbohydrates, starches, grains, breads, flesh proteins, dill pickles, preserved luncheon meats, frozen vegetables, and canned meats. She was deficient in these quality sodium foods: kelp, olives, cheddar cheese, scallops, cottage cheese, lobster, Swiss chard, beets and greens, buttermilk, and celery. She took herbs for her type, started exercising, and her weight steadily decreased as she returned to her figure of twenty years ago. Her emotional state became more stable.

————

Desmogenic Type Mineral Needs

Apply this mineral data to the diet following the Muscle type descriptions.

Excessive Foods:

- *Sodium (salted, junk) speed*
- *Carbon (simple carbohydrates)*
- *Nitrogen (beef)*

Deficient Foods:

- *Sodium (unsalted, non-junk))*
- *Chloride (unsalted)*
- *Nitrogen (non-beef, vegetable)*
- *Potassium*
- *Phosphorus*
- *Silicon*
- *Magnesium*

These deficient nutrients are common deficiencies in your type, and predispose you to ill-health.
If ill, be sure to use these lists with your <u>daily</u> food intake. If not ill, eat from the food lists 3-4 days <u>weekly</u> for health maintenance. All food lists are in descending order of concentration and value to you; choose servings of foods in the upper half of each list first! One serving is ½ cup.

Desmogenic Excessive Foods –

Sodium from salted junk foods is excessive in your tissues (more than in any other type) and propels you into disease; it is the major cause of your common arthritis and connective tissue diseases. To preserve your health and weight control avoid junk; fulfill your sodium needs from the food list (<u>without</u> the salt shaker).

▶ *Rocine: "Inorganic sodium (salt) often predominates in your diet leading to arthritis, arterial hardening, and disease. You usually eat too much beef, a major cause of your health problems."*

Carbon is excessive in your type and should be minimized. It is excessive in all people who become fat or obese, and is found in every cell of the body as the basis of life.

Nitrogen from red meat is excessive in your diet (if eaten more than 1-2 times monthly after age 30-40), and is a major cause of your acidity and illnesses; poultry, fish and eggs should be taken about four days weekly, with vegetarian proteins like legumes (peas, beans), seeds, nuts and pasta on the other days. (After age 50, some of you choose vegetarianism, which helps your healing and graceful aging.)

———

Deficient Foods -

In illness or disease, it is important to correct these mineral deficiencies.

Sodium foods are deficient in your type (see above note).

Chloride is deficient in your tissues. Found in all cells and tissues, it is particularly active in the health of your pancreas, stomach, cartilage, sexual organs, lymph, and blood.

Nitrogen from vegetable sources is deficient (see above note).

Potassium is deficient in your type. It is concentrated in and vital to the health of your muscles, heart, brain, and all cells. If you are ill or diseased, potassium foods and supplements are invariably an important healing and anti-arthritic factor.

Phosphorus is often deficient in your tissues, and is needed because of intense nervous system activity and brain exhaustion. You are always thinking, planning, and worrying about everything in your life—especially your health.

Silicon is invariably deficient in your tissues, and eating such foods is essential for your connective tissue health (especially if you have arthritis or other diseases).

Magnesium is often deficient in your type, and is particularly important for your heart and digestive function; deficiency links to diabetes, migraines, osteoporosis, heart disease, and high blood pressure.

Pure vegetarianism is unhealthy for you before age 40-50! If determined to do it, be sure to take about 30 gm. of a protein drink daily (and find a good doctor)! You require a variety of vegetarianism where you eat liberally of proteins and complex carbohydrates (acidifying).

Note –

The food recommendations are for the generic type. Additionally, you may need from a holistic healer or nutritionist something more specific for your individuality.

———

<u>*Minimize*</u>
Excessive Foods

Sodium (salted, junk): *0-2 servings/week*

Salt, all fast foods, packaged foods, canned and frozen foods, soy sauce, all preserved meats (cured, smoked, canned and luncheon meats), sauces (barbecue, catsup, etc.), dill pickles, sauerkraut, bouillon cubes, peanut butter, potato chips, etc., salted nuts, crackers, canned or packaged soups, processed cheeses, commercial salad dressings, meat tenderizer. [Lose the salt shaker!]
Note: If you must eat anything on the above list, keep it down to ½ cup, 0-2 times weekly!

Carbon: *2-3 servings/week*

Simple carbohydrates, dairy foods, white bread, sweet fruits, simple sugars

Nitrogen (beef):

Beef, red meats: 0-2 times/ <u>**month**</u>

Eat
Deficient Foods

Sodium, Chloride (non-junk):
1-2 servings/day

Kelp, fish, milk, cheese, olives, cottage cheese, gizzard, lentils, almonds, lobster, Swiss chard, beets and greens, buttermilk, celery (and juice), spinach, chicken.

Potassium, Silicon: *1-2 servings/day*

Dulse, kelp, blackstrap molasses, strawberries, alfalfa, brewers yeast, rice bran, whole grains, sunflower seeds, almonds, raisins, parsley, sesame seeds, rice polish, dried prunes, peanuts, soybean, Swiss chard, herbs (oat straw, horsetail).

Phosphorus, Magnesium:
1-2 servings/day

Kelp, whole wheat, seeds, nuts, blackstrap molasses, brewer's yeast, soybeans, pinto beans (dried), buckwheat, dulse, grains, rye, barley.

Nitrogen (non-beef, vegetable):

Legumes, peas, cabbage, black-eyed peas, seeds, most nuts, pasta, spirulina, oranges, potatoes, soybeans —as desired

Eggs, poultry, fish —3-4 times weekly

Note: Eat any healthy foods you desire, but be sure to include the type foods in your daily choices.

Desmogenic Nutritional Supplements

- **Multi-Vitamins** —
  [Take all supplements with food]
  2 capsules/day
- **Potassium** —
  About 200 mg/day with food
- **Do not take extra Calcium**
  [You absorb it excessively.]
  (Exception: stress, menopause, osteoporosis, or if on estrogen)
- **Magnesium** —
  200 mg/day with food
- **Herbs** —
  Brain detox – Chickweed or Valerian Root
  Organ detox – Echinacea Root or Red Clover
  (Take one capsule, twice daily for one month; then one capsule, three times weekly.)
- **Lecithin** —
  About 1,300 mg/three times weekly
- **Evening Primrose or Flaxseed Oil** —
  1 soft-gel/day

Important Desmogenic Health Concerns

Your nervous system genetics require the carnivorous *Muscle* type food guide for health, and any flesh cravings are normal and healthy for you. After about age 50, you need less flesh, a *semi-vegetarian* diet being preferred with about four flesh days and three vegetarian days weekly.

Some of you choose vegetarianism and should be careful to obtain sufficient daily protein—you need more protein than the average person. Take a daily powdered protein drink as a supplement (about 30 gm.), in addition to your protein foods. You need an *acid-ash* vegetarian diet (as below).

Like the *calciferic* type you tend to over-eat flesh, especially beef, calcium, pasteurized cheese and dairy foods until diseased. Potassium foods and salads, twice daily, help to moderate your acidity from excessive flesh and protein intake.

<u>*DESMOGENIC FOOD GUIDE*</u>

Aim for -
50% Proteins, complex carbohydrates
50% Fruits, salads, vegetables
and
50% Raw food diet
50% Cooked foods

<u>**Lose the salt shaker!**</u>
<u>**Minimize beef and all dairy foods.**</u>
Follow the Mineral Food recommendations.
Take the recommended supplements.

Desmogenic Weight Loss

Weight problems are commonly developed after age 30-40, particularly if a fat sub-type is present. Losing weight depends upon you following the type instructions, summarized in this section:

- *Stop* eating junk sodium and carbon foods (see lists)
- *Have a protein* drink daily, about 25-30 grams
- *Eat* your body type deficient mineral foods daily

- *Follow* your *Desmogenic Food Guide* instructions
- *Exercise:* your body type requires strong, intense exercise daily!
- *Simple sugars:* stop all white table sugar and high-fructose corn syrup and drinks containing these sugars
- *Calories:* As with any dietary approach, calories in, must be *less than* calories out! Most markets sell a calorie booklet; make notes of your daily intake, and in most instances keep it under about 1500 calories/day

———

Muscle Types
General Food Guide
(Carnivores)

Important Note

The Food Guide addresses the <u>Acid-Alkaline</u> aspect of your food intake, along with the <u>Type Mineral</u> factor presented throughout this book. It does <u>not</u> necessarily address calories or other dietary factors that may be pertinent to your personal health needs whether medical or appropriate for some other dietary need. So use your common sense and just include the factors described here with whatever healthy dietary choices you usually make.

For other nutrient information, consult with nutritional books or with holistic nutritional doctors. In this regard, I particularly recommend the advice of Andrew Weil, M.D.

Muscle Types
General Food Guide

(Not for the Nitropheric Type)

This chapter presents a general Food Guide, upon which you superimpose the nutritional information from your type chapter. As a Muscle body type your genetics require flesh foods.

Meat/Flesh Intake

Most muscle types should limit red meat to once or less weekly, while eggs, lamb, fish, or poultry are excellent in moderation. If ill or diseased, be sure to eat daily, one or two servings from each *deficient minerals* list. If not ill, eat them at least three times weekly for health maintenance. If this diet is similar to your present diet, but healing is sluggish, then:

- Decrease your carbohydrate and protein intake by about one-third
- Increase your fruit, salad, and vegetable intake by about one-third
- Consult with a holistic doctor, preferably one versed in nutritional and emotional evaluation

---

Over-Acid or Over-Alkaline?

Just as a log of wood burned in your fireplace leaves a mineral-ash, food ash refers to the minerals remaining after metabolizing foods in your tissues:

- Fruits, vegetables **alkalinize** tissues
- Proteins, carbohydrates **acidify** tissues

Usually You Are Over-Acid Due To:

- Excessive intake of dairy foods
- Excessive intake of proteins and carbohydrates
- Deficient intake of fruits, salads and vegetables
- Accumulated metabolic waste-acids (from years of eating excessive acid-ash foods, meats and carbohydrates, and from lack of exercise)
- You need to estimate the ratio of foods eaten. Generally, eat the following *approximate* ratios for your health:

50% <u>**Alkaline-ash**</u> foods *(fruits, salads, vegetables)*

50% <u>**Acid-ash**</u> foods *(complex carbohydrates like starches, grains, cereals, breads, flour products; and proteins)*

Approximate your food ratios. On any particular day, it does not matter if one meal is mostly alkaline, and another mostly acid—just try to balance it out for the day! If you get it wrong, try again tomorrow. It is a subjective call that you make, and it is what you do over weeks, months, or years that make the difference—not on any one or two days.

––––––

If Vegetarian

As a general indication, if you follow a vegetarian diet substitute vegetable sources of protein for the any flesh in the food guide. Note that contrary to most alkaline-ash vegetarian diets you need something different:

*You need an **acid-ash** vegetarian diet high in complex carbohydrates and vegetable proteins.*

Because of your high need for protein, you usually require a vegetable powdered protein supplement in juice (about 25-30 grams daily).

––––––

Important

- Minimize white sugar and alcohol intake.
- If desired, interchange lunches for dinners.

- Never eat foods you are allergic to, no matter what I recommend; if allergic, or suspect a food allergy, eliminate it and substitute from your type mineral lists.
- Eat the right foods 80-90% of the time and the Food Guide will work for you; unlike some types you do not have to live out of a health food store (although such foods are healthier for you).

▶ *Omit eating the excessive minerals in your type chapter, and be sure to eat one or two servings from the deficient list daily.*

Finally, in addition to your body type needs, other holistic healing matters also need your attention. I strongly suggest that you refer to my web site and earlier books for that information: *DrStenbeck.net*

———

Acid/Alkaline Genetics Chart

The following chart reflects each Muscle Type and its acid or alkaline-ash food needs. These ratios change if you are unhealthy or over age 45-50. Refer back to your body type and review the *Acid/alkaline* instructions.

———

Acid/Alkaline Genetics, Dietary-Ash, and Raw Food Needs

This chart shows the Rocine types, their acid or alkaline food needs, and the percentage of raw foods needed for your health and healing.

- Apply your Type Minerals to the Food Guide

Type	Acid/Alkaline Genetics	% Food-Ash Needed	% Raw Food Needed
Calciferic	Alkaline	70% acid	30
Carbogenic	Alkaline	50-50	50
Desmogenic	Alkaline	70% acid	50
Eldic	Intermediate	50-50	50
Medeic	Intermediate	50-50	50
Myogenic	Intermediate	50-50	50
Nervimotive	Alkaline	70% acid	50
Nitropheric	Acid	70% alkaline	70
Pallinomic	Alkaline	50-50	30

The above percentages vary depending on aging and the health of individual types.

Muscle Types / Food Guide
<u>*Breakfast*</u>

[Superimpose the nutritional information from your

EGGS (1-2) with lettuce, tomato, or salad, whole grain toast; (add bacon or sausage 1-3 times weekly if desired)
— 2-4 times/week; or*

*FRUIT fresh salad, and protein (yogurt, milk, cheeses, seeds, nuts)
—1-3 times/week; or*

*CEREALS, with fruit, seeds, nuts
—2-5 times/week; or*

*OTHER choices
— 0-1 times weekly*

<u>*Daily liquids:*</u>
*Pure water, citrus, vegetable juices, soups, other —as desired
Coffee, teas —0-2 cups*

[Include selections from your type mineral needs everyday.]

Muscle Types / Food Guide

<u>Lunch</u>

SALADS, mixed green, protein
(poultry, fish, egg, cheese, seeds or nuts,
etc.), whole grain breads
 [Dressing: olive oil/ vinegar; low-fat, low-
 cal dressings]
— 2-4 times/ week; or

SANDWICH, whole grains with a
protein (cheese, tuna, ham, etc.); and salad
and/ or vegetables
— 1-4 times/ week; or

POULTRY, FISH, 3-6 oz., with a
mixed green salad and/ or vegetables
—1-3 times/ week; or

OTHER choices (with salad or vegetables)
—1-2 times/ week

[Other oils permitted, but less ideal is
soybean oil, a common allergen; minimize
commercial dressings. Be sure to include two or
more selections from your type food lists in your
daily food intake. For in-between meal snacks,
eat fruit or vegetables with seeds/ nuts.]

[Include selections from your type mineral
needs everyday.]

Muscle Types / Food Guide
Dinner

POULTRY, FISH *(4-6 oz.), with salad and/ or vegetables*
—2-4 times/week; or

PASTA *with protein (chicken, etc.) with salad and/ or vegetables*
— 2-4 times/week; or

VEGETARIAN *meal with salad and/ or vegetables*
—1-3 times/week; or

LEAN BEEF *(4-6 oz.) with salad and/ or vegetables*
— 0-1 times/week

OTHER *choices with salad and/ or vegetables*
— 0-1 times/week

Desserts:
Fruits, fresh —as desired
Low-sugar, healthy desserts
— 0-3 times/wk
[Include selections from your type mineral needs everyday.]

Food Guide Notes

Steamed Vegetables —

Minerals are lost in the boiling of vegetables; steaming or wok cooking is best.

Food Combinations —

If you have a weak digestive system then eating proteins at the same meal with starches often results in indigestion, gas, or constipation.

Periodic Detox —

You tend to over-indulge in acid-ash foods (proteins and carbohydrates), and often need occasional elimination diets for tissue waste-acid removal. Have a holistic doctor or nutritionist supervise such detox (where you have an alkaline-ash diet along with protein supplementation).

Minimize —

- Fatty foods
- Commercial salad dressings
- Beef, red meats, processed meats
- Coffee, white sugar, corn syrup, alcohol

Vegetarian Proteins —

You require a carnivorous diet. An exception is the *nitropheric* type who functions best with a *vegetarian* diet. The other muscle types are born to be carnivores. It is very difficult for the other muscle types to be pure vegetarians because of their strong intuitive cravings for fish, poultry, meat, or eggs. If you are vegetarian, then because of your high needs for amino acids and acid-ash foods, you should take a protein supplement of 30-40 grams/day (powdered protein in juice).

Healthy Weight —

Several of you gain weight as the ravages of age, lack of exercise and dietary excesses take their toll. By eating according to your body type, you should naturally lose excess weight. Each type also has a few individual factors that only apply to them!

You have a good ability to lose weight by following the Food Guide instructions. The most common problem I find with your weight-control is liver and kidney irritation due to food allergies, which results in extra pounds. The key is to eat non-allergic foods.

If drinking more than 3-4 cups daily of coffee or tea, you may have a hypoglycemic problem (low blood sugar), which contributes to making fat, ill-health, and delayed healing. (Refer to the earlier books for help with this healing.)

———

Appendix

Brief Extracts from
The 22 Unique Body Types

Appendix A

Types
(Brief extract)

Type comes from 'typus' meaning an image or impression, the study of types being called typology.

► *Rocine: "A combination of mental and structural features is consistently found in people of the same type."*

Rocine wrote that all types are a mixture of positive and negative qualities. He based his work on the biochemical individuality of our *mineral* absorption and utilization. Of course, all minerals are absorbed, but he postulated that different types of people *selectively* absorb certain minerals, to a greater or lesser extent, requiring specific mineral foods for their enhanced health and healing.

► *The type information cannot predict what or who you will become, or how successful or not, but your type is capable of bringing a creative excellence to whatever you do in life. If your type has negative qualities that you disagree with, remember that they are only tendencies and may or may not manifest in you.*

This book enlarges on Rocine's premise (early 1900's), integrated with the later research of Herbert Sheldon, M.D., Ph.D., at Harvard University (1930's), along with my fifty years of observations and experience with this subject.

Comparing your shared physical (and sometimes psychological) descriptions with the Celebrity Lists further assists the identification of your type. It is not that you will look exactly like, or be a twin to, any particular celebrity. Look closely at a celebrity's features: face, profile, height, weight, head, etc. If you know something about their talents, beliefs, success and failure spheres, health and weight challenges, attitudes and behaviors, etc., then you get clues as to what your type may be.

Understanding Types and Sub-Types

Each of us has a clearly discernible dominant type. Visualize the celebrity examples from movies, politics, sports, the arts and public life, and try to identify with their physical features. Look for similar features, remembering that you will not recognize all attributes in yourself. You are not looking for your twin!

The sub-type issue is the main reason people of the same major type can look so different. Remember that a type description does not characterize you exactly, but depicts your individual variant of a type.

► *The type questionnaire pinpoints the major features of that type: if the celebrity examples are unhelpful, you may be an unusual variant (in which case ignore the celebrity issue and give yourself 7 points on Question 1).*

Minerals

Minerals are essential life nutrients that accelerate enzyme and chemical reactions and provide a basis for your body typing. Although found in all tissues, different minerals tend to be concentrated in certain organs, their presence or absence contributing to the healing of such tissues; e.g., zinc accelerates prostate healing; calcium and manganese promote bone, joint and connective tissue healing.

Specific foods nurture each type, some people needing meats for their health others needing a vegetarian diet. A high potassium diet nurtures one person, while another needs high sulfur, calcium, zinc, or another mineral.

Mineral Digestion and Absorption

Compared to vitamins, minerals are *difficult* to digest, absorb, and utilize. In people with strong digestive systems, this aspect may not be important. The following factors should be in place for optimal mineral metabolism:

1. Stomach Hydrochloric Acid Production
2. Parathyroid Hormone Balance
3. Organ Toxic Metal and Chemical Removal
   [See details in <u>The 22 Unique Body Types.</u>]

———

Total Body Healing

Note that from a holistic healing perspective, in addition to minerals and type information, the following healing factors are necessary:

> *Nutrient Balance*
> *Mental Balance*
> *Emotional Balance*
> *Spiritual Balance*
> *Detoxifying Integrity*

The above factors are all important to your total healing especially if you are interested in self-healing (see my earlier books).

———

Appendix B

Researchers
(Brief extract)

The predominant workers in this area of human individuality from around 1880's to the 1960's are Herbert Sheldon, M.D., Ph.D., Roger Williams, Ph.D., and Victor Rocine, D.Sc.

Much information on Sheldon's research exists on-line and in medical psychology libraries; for interested readers there are other lines of research published in the last century. This present book is primarily about Rocine's body types.

Herbert Sheldon M.D., Ph.D.

In contrast to Rocine, Sheldon at Harvard University in the 1930's was trained in the scientific method and did painstaking research and publishing on human individuality. In comparing his findings with Rocine's work, a direct putative correlation is visible.

Roger J. Williams, Ph.D.

Another significant researcher in human individuality is the renowned scientist and biochemist, Roger J. Williams. He demonstrated that different people have varying levels of nutrients, enzymes, and other metabolic chemicals in their bloodstreams.

▶ *Williams's research firmly expands on the premise of individual nutritional needs in human beings. If interested in his research, I highly recommend his book Biochemial Individuality.*

Victor Rocine, D.Sc.

Note that when a negative feature is indicated, say neurotic tendencies, all members of the type are <u>not</u> that way; it is a type tendency reported by Rocine.

Rocine studied type-related diseases finding links between mineral and dietary factors with individual types and their diseases. In each body type, one or more dominant minerals are preferentially absorbed and utilized over other minerals.

He recognized discrete body types from their physical appearance finding genetically based mineral dominance to be the determining feature. He also correlated their physical features with psychological characteristics.

Genetics, Types, and Diet
(Brief extract)

This section deals with how nervous system genetics helps determine your eating choices for health: you are either born to be a predominant meat eater, a partial or complete vegetarian, or something between the two. The genetic factor determining this dietary aspect is the *sympathetic and parasympathetic* components of your central nervous system. This represents a basic factor in eating for health.

This chapter helps you understand your dietary inheritance, although instinctively, you may already have arrived there!

- If born **sympathetic** dominant you are *genetically acid*, desiring a predominantly *vegetarian* diet for your health (about 70% fruit, salad, vegetables to 30% proteins and carbohydrates).

- If born **parasympathetic** dominant you are *genetically alkaline*, desiring a predominantly *carnivorous* diet for your health (about 70% proteins, carbohydrates to 30% fruits, salads, vegetables). Few of you ever choose to become vegetarian because of the difficulty in satisfying your protein needs without meats.

- If born ***intermediate*** dominant you may eat food groups with little concern for the acid/alkaline factor. However, after age 40, you need a semi-vegetarian diet for healthy eating.

———

Chart of Relative Nervous System Dominance

In the following Chart, if you relate to many of the symptoms on one side you probably have that nervous system dominance; relating to both sides indicates *Intermediate* dominance.

If Vegetarian (Over-acid) --
> *Eat 70% fruits, salads, vegetables*
> *And 30% proteins, carbohydrates*

If Carnivore (Over-alkaline) --
> *Eat 70% proteins, carbohydrates*
> *And 30% fruits, salads, vegetables*

If Intermediate --
> *Eat 50:50 of acid and alkaline-ash foods*

Make an *approximate* estimate of your daily acid and alkaline food intake (such ratios varying from type to type).

———

Symptoms of Relative Genetic Dominance

Vegetarians (Over-acid)	Carnivores (Over-alkaline)
Sympathetic Dominance	*Parasympathetic Dominance*
little or no flesh desire	desire flesh
easily constipated	rarely constipated
slow digestion	fast digestion
easily dehydrated	not dehydrated
strong thirst	low thirst
pale face	flushed face
high pulse after food	slow pulse after food
easy gag reflex	slow gag reflex
cool dry skin	moist warm skin
nervous stomach	calm stomach
little eyelid blinking	much blinking
nervous tendency	mostly calm
slower healing	faster healing
low oxygen-uptake	good oxygen-uptake
easily breathless	seldom breathless
insomnia common	sleep easier
few muscle cramps	some night cramps
calcium deposits rare	get calcium deposits

Appendix D

Help Identifying your Body Type with Dr. Stenbeck

If you desire help in identifying your body type, follow these instructions, and answer the questionnaire. For further information and fees, send me an email from page one of the website:

DrStenbeck.net

First name: ________________

Country of birth: ________________

Upload photos and send to the above website:

- Head and shoulders: front and side views

- Full body: front and side views

- Also 1-2 teenage views

- If possible, casual photos of mother, father, siblings

MY TYPE CLASS MAY BE: ____________

(Thin, Muscle, or Fat)

AGE - _______

HEIGHT - _______ feet/inches

MY WEIGHT - _______ pounds

Heaviest at age: _______

- Lightest as adult: ___________

- Estimate age 15: ___________

VISION - Excellent Average   Poor:

HAIR - Natural color: ___________

- Thin/thick? ___________

- balding? ___________

SKIN - Quality: ___________

- History of acne, boils, other:

____

____

TEETH   - Strong   Weak   Dentures

- Cavity history: Many   Moderate Few

MUSCLES - Strong   Average   Weak

Sports played _________________________

JOINTS   - Strong   Average   Weak

HEALTH - Childhood diseases?

____

____

- Adult diseases?

____

AVERAGE DIET

- Beef ___________ (times/week)

- Poultry ___________ (times/week)

- Fish ___________ (times/week)

- Eggs ___________ (times/week)

- Water ___________ (glasses/day):

- Vegetarian? Vegan? ___________

- Other? ___________________________

- Did your childhood diet differ? _______

The above will help me know who you are! I will send you a follow-up questionnaire for further help in identifying your body type.

Appendix E

On-line Health Consultation with Dr. Stenbeck

For further information, or to comment on this book, or to receive a response on any health issue from a holistic viewpoint, send an email inquiry from page one of my website:

DrStenbeck.net

Following that, I will suggest further healing needs, which we may pursue with an on-line consult.

———

Appendix F

Notes

See my book *The 22 Unique Body Types,* available at the usual online source, for further information and details on all of the 22 Types. The Appendix in that book has further information about:

Mineral Functions and Food Sources

Further Reading

———